MAKE-UP

Felicity Everett

Illustrated by Conny Jude

Consultant: Saskia Sarginson

Designed by Camilla Luff

Edited by Angela Wilkes

CONTENTS

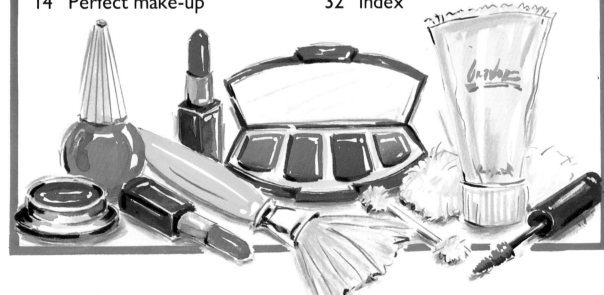

About this book

Make-up is exciting and colourful. You can wear as much, or as little, as you like. The important thing is to wear make-up which suits you and is right for the occasion.

This book shows you how to choose and put on make-up. It also gives you lots of ideas for ways to vary the basic looks in the book and invent some of your own.

Your make-up kit

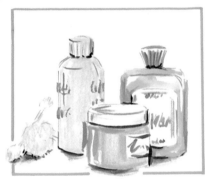

Before you begin to experiment with make-up, you need to collect your make-up kit.

A few simple items go a long way. You can find out which basic things you need on pages 8-9.

Skincare

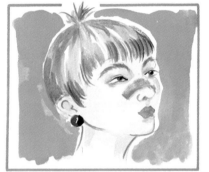

You can find out what kind of skin you have, and how to look after it on pages 4-5.

A daily cleansing routine

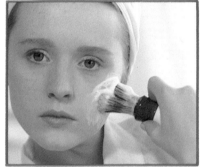

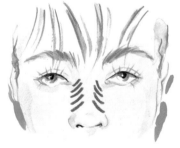

A really effective cleansing routine is important if you wear make-up. On pages 6-7, there is a daily cleansing routine you can follow, and a table telling you which products suit your skin.

Choosing colours

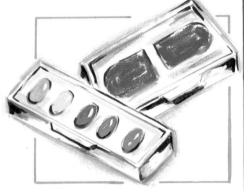

Turn to page 10 for some hints on which make-up shades might flatter your colouring.

Shaping and shading with colours

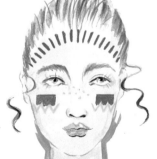

You can use highlighter, shader and blusher to make your face look more oval, to disguise a double chin, or to 'slim' your nose. You can find out how to do it on page 12.

A perfect make-up

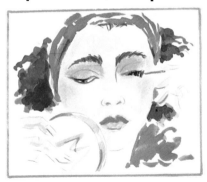

The make-up techniques in this book are illustrated step-by-step so you know exactly what to do.

Handy hints

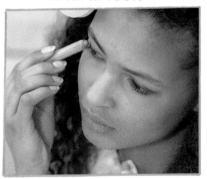

Pictures in boxes this shape and size give tips on how to apply your make-up better.

The natural look

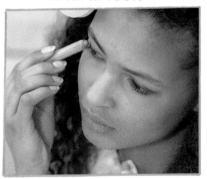

On page 18, you can find out how to do a natural-looking make-up, with the minimum of fuss.

Top-to-toe beauty treatment

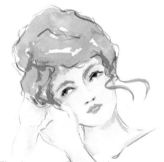

The beauty routine on pages 20-23 includes conditioning treatments for your hair.

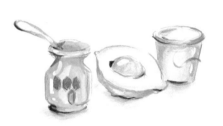

There are also recipes for home-made face masks using natural ingredients.

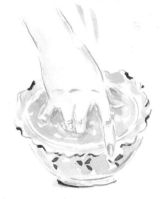

You can see how to give your hands a manicure and there are lots more ideas too.

Bright ideas for party make-up

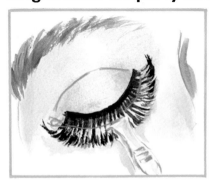

From page 24 onwards, you will find some colourful and original ideas for party make-up.

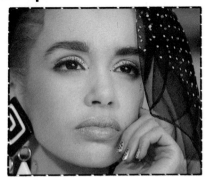

The step-by-step instructions are as detailed as before, but the results are more dramatic.

Nostalgic looks

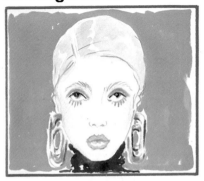

On pages 30-31, you can find out how to re-create nostalgic make-up looks from the past.

Looking after your skin

It is important to look after your skin properly, especially if you wear make-up.

To keep it healthy, you should cleanse and moisturise it each day. You will need:

Cleanser is cream or lotion which you use to clean your skin and take off your make-up. You can see how to do it on pages 6-7.

Moisturiser is cream or lotion which protects and softens your skin and stops it from becoming too dry. You can see how to put it on over the page.

Toner is liquid which closes up the pores after you have cleansed your skin and freshens it.

You can use a **cleansing bar** instead of cleanser, if your skin is oily. This looks like ordinary soap, but will not dry your skin.

Eye make-up remover can be liquid, or ready-to-use pads. It removes eye make-up gently.

Cotton buds are good for touching your face without making it greasy.

Cotton wool and tissues are useful for taking off your make-up and for putting on creams and lotions.

Diet

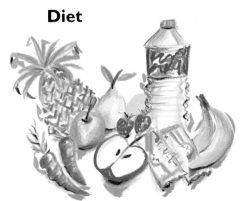

For clear healthy skin, eat plenty of fresh fruit and vegetables and drink lots of water. Don't eat sweets.

What skin type are you?

Look for skin care products which are recommended for your type of skin. If you don't know what type yours is, the simple test below will tell you whether your skin is dry, oily or normal. All you need is a roll of sticky tape.

Press a piece of sticky tape lightly over the bridge of your nose and on to your cheeks, avoiding the area round your eyes. Pull it off and look at it.

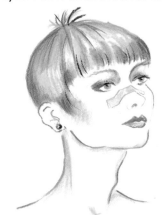

white flakes = dry skin
drops of moisture = oily skin
both = normal skin

Problem skin

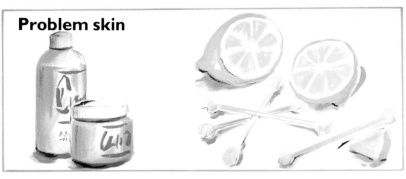

If you often get rashes, look for hypo-allergenic products. They are made from pure ingredients which should not irritate your skin.

If you get lots of spots, use medicated skin products. *Never* squeeze spots. If you have a bad one, dab it gently with a cotton bud soaked in lemon juice.

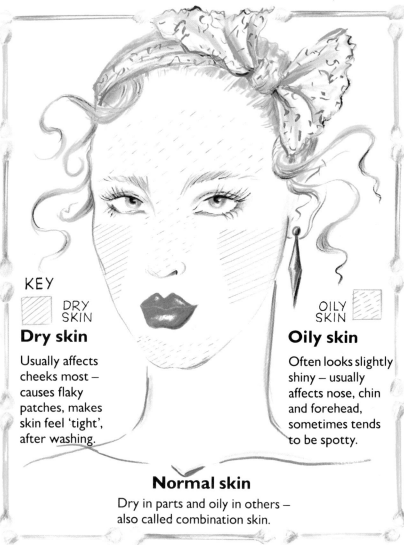

KEY

DRY SKIN

OILY SKIN

Dry skin

Usually affects cheeks most – causes flaky patches, makes skin feel 'tight', after washing.

Oily skin

Often looks slightly shiny – usually affects nose, chin and forehead, sometimes tends to be spotty.

Normal skin

Dry in parts and oily in others – also called combination skin.

Cleansing

Follow this simple cleansing routine every morning* and evening.

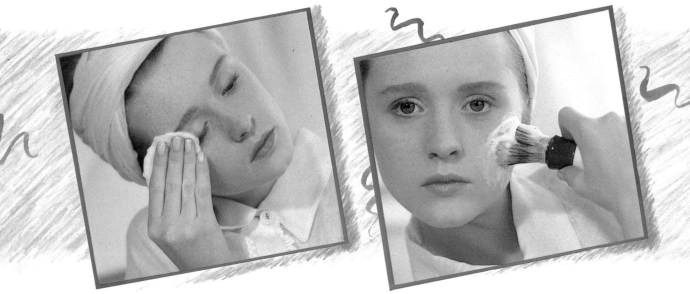

1   Removing eye make-up

Apply make-up remover with cotton wool. Gently stroke it downwards and inwards towards the corner of each eye, making sure you do not pull the skin around your eyes.

2   Cleansing

If you use a cleansing bar, lather your face with a shaving brush, then rinse it off. Or you can smooth cream cleanser over your face and neck, then wipe it off gently with a tissue.

Finding the right products for your skin

This chart shows you which creams and lotions suit different types of skin.

To find out what type of skin you have, do the simple test on page 5.

Skin type	Cleanser	Toner	Moisturiser
Dry skin	Cream or thick liquid cleanser.	Mild toner: camomile, rose water, or still mineral water.	cream moisturiser.
Oily skin	Lotion or cleansing milk.	Natural astringent, such as witch hazel or cucumber.	Light, non-greasy liquid moisturiser.
Combination skin	Creamy liquid or cream cleanser.	Mild toner: camomile, rosewater or still mineral water.	Thin cream or thick lotion.

* You will not need to remove eye make-up in the morning.

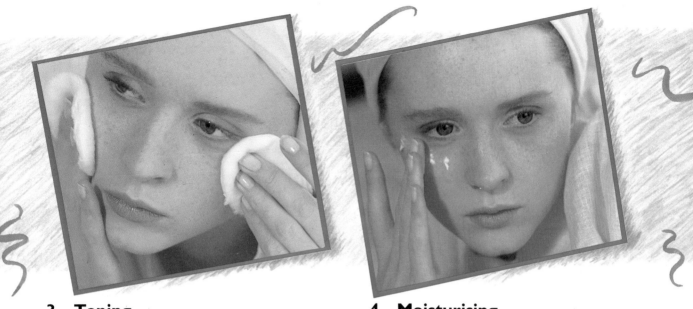

3 Toning

Soak a cotton wool pad in toner and gently wipe it over your face. Or you can put the toner into an atomiser (an old, clean perfume spray would do) and spray it over your face.

4 Moisturising

Put little dots of moisturiser over your face and neck and gently rub it into your skin with your fingertips. You can put more on areas which are especially dry, such as your cheeks.

Deep cleansing

Deep cleansing about once a fortnight helps to keep your skin soft and really clean.

Any of the methods shown below work well. Used together, they make an excellent facial.

Facial sauna

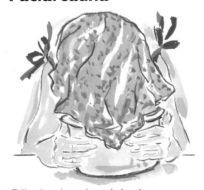

Fill a big bowl with boiling water. Hold your face about 20cm from the water and drape a towel over your head to stop steam from escaping. Wait for five minutes.

Facial scrubs

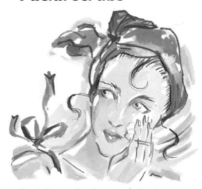

Facial scrubs (or exfoliating creams) contain tiny granules which rub off the top layer of skin. Read the instructions on the packet for what to do.

Face masks*

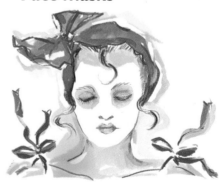

You can buy gels, creams, or mud-based masks. Choose one which is recommended for your type of skin. Read the instructions on the packet for what to do.

* You will find some recipes for home-made face masks on page 21.

Your make-up kit

Here are the things you need to do a complete make-up, like the one on pages 14-17.

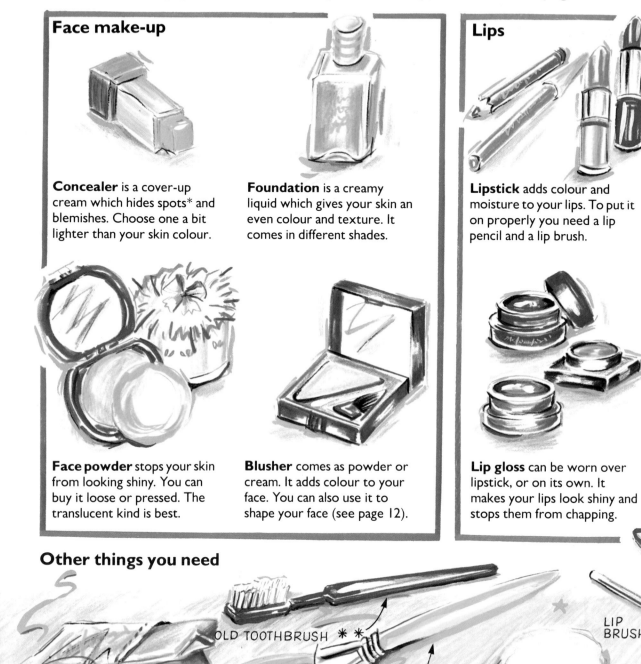

Face make-up

Concealer is a cover-up cream which hides spots* and blemishes. Choose one a bit lighter than your skin colour.

Foundation is a creamy liquid which gives your skin an even colour and texture. It comes in different shades.

Face powder stops your skin from looking shiny. You can buy it loose or pressed. The translucent kind is best.

Blusher comes as powder or cream. It adds colour to your face. You can also use it to shape your face (see page 12).

Lips

Lipstick adds colour and moisture to your lips. To put it on properly you need a lip pencil and a lip brush.

Lip gloss can be worn over lipstick, or on its own. It makes your lips look shiny and stops them from chapping.

Other things you need

TISSUES

OLD TOOTHBRUSH **

POWDER BRUSH

POWDER PUFF

LIP BRUSH

Make-up often comes with its own brushes and applicators, but for a really professional look, you will need to collect some tools of your own. Here are some useful ones to start off with.

8   * You can buy medicated concealer especially for spots.   ** For combing your eyebrows.

Eye make-up

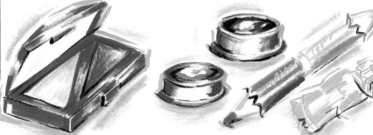

Eye-shadows come in different forms. To start with, choose two matching pressed powder eye-shadows.

You can also buy eye-shadow in pots (of powder or cream), in tubes (of cream), or in pencils (of powder or cream).

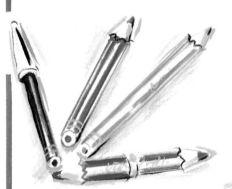

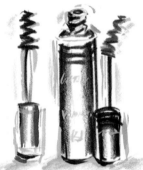

Eye pencil is for outlining your eyes, close to your eyelashes. Choose one a shade darker than your eye-shadow.

Mascara is thick liquid for darkening your eyelashes, you put it on with a brush. Use black or brown for everyday.

Professional make-up tips

Do not lend your make-up to anyone, even your best friend. You can pass on eye infections and cold sores.

To check that your foundation is the right colour for you, test it on your face (without any make-up on).

Keep your pencils sharp. You can sharpen them better if you put them in the fridge for an hour before you need them.

Keep your make-up in a clean, dry place. A box with compartments, such as a plastic tool box is ideal.

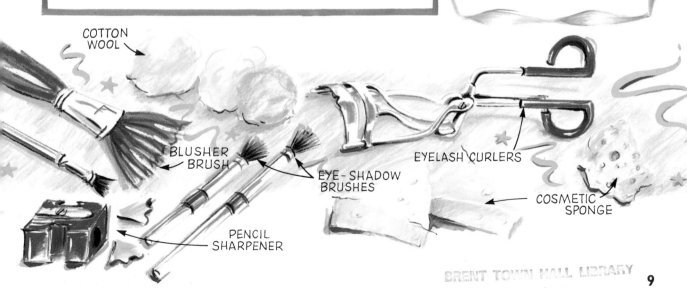

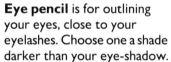

COTTON WOOL

BLUSHER BRUSH

EYE-SHADOW BRUSHES

EYELASH CURLERS

COSMETIC SPONGE

PENCIL SHARPENER

Choosing colours

It is fun trying out make-up colours, but mistakes can be expensive. It is best to choose shades which go with your colouring.

Here are six typical hair and skin colours. Below each picture, you can see the make-up colours which flatter that type.

Fair skin/brown hair

Brunettes often have fair skin and rosy cheeks. If your skin looks blotchy, even it out with a creamy-beige foundation.

Fair skin/blonde hair

Blondes have fair, rather dry skin which needs careful skin care. Use a pinkish foundation to give colour to your skin.

Freckled skin/red hair

Redheads tend to have fair, sensitive, freckled skin. Choose a light foundation which lets your freckles show through.

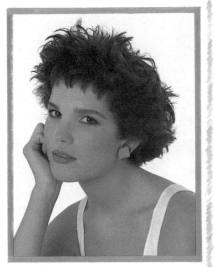

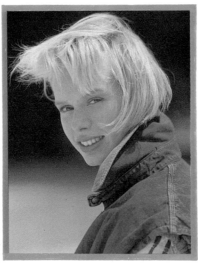

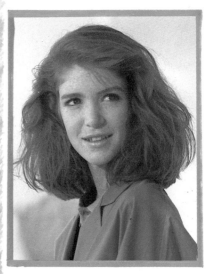

Blusher

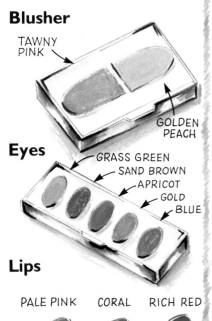

TAWNY PINK

GOLDEN PEACH

Eyes

GRASS GREEN
SAND BROWN
APRICOT
GOLD
BLUE

Lips

PALE PINK   CORAL   RICH RED

Blusher

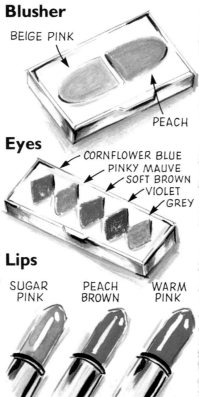

BEIGE PINK

PEACH

Eyes

CORNFLOWER BLUE
PINKY MAUVE
SOFT BROWN
VIOLET
GREY

Lips

SUGAR PINK   PEACH BROWN   WARM PINK

Blusher

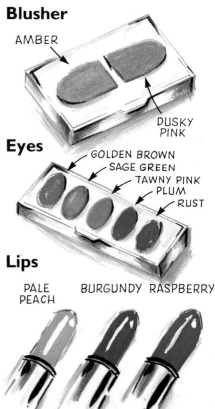

AMBER

DUSKY PINK

Eyes

GOLDEN BROWN
SAGE GREEN
TAWNY PINK
PLUM
RUST

Lips

PALE PEACH   BURGUNDY   RASPBERRY

Several companies make foundations and concealers especially for dark skin. You can mix two colours together if you cannot find the right shade.

Do not wear powder. It will just make your skin look dull. Let it's natural sheen show through a light coating of foundation.

Black skin/dark hair

Black skin can be oily and sometimes the colour is a little uneven. Even it out with a light, non-greasy foundation.

Brown skin/dark hair

Brown skin can be slightly blotchy. Mix foundation and concealer and then use the mixture to even out your colouring.

Olive skin/dark hair

Olive skin can look sallow and may be oily, but a non-greasy, dark beige foundation can make it look healthy and golden.

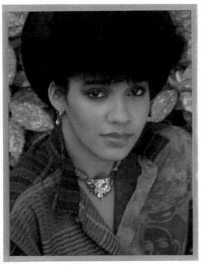

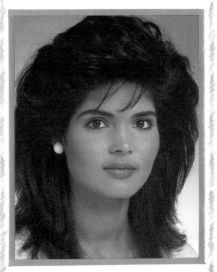

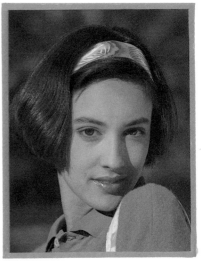

Blusher

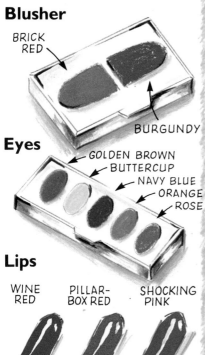

BRICK RED

BURGUNDY

Blusher

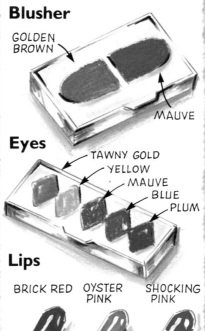

GOLDEN BROWN

MAUVE

Blusher

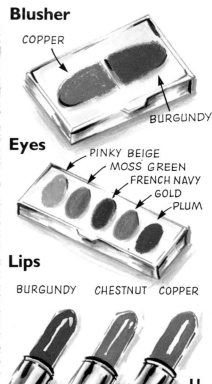

COPPER

BURGUNDY

Eyes

GOLDEN BROWN
BUTTERCUP
NAVY BLUE
ORANGE
ROSE

Eyes

TAWNY GOLD
YELLOW
MAUVE
BLUE
PLUM

Eyes

PINKY BEIGE
MOSS GREEN
FRENCH NAVY
GOLD
PLUM

Lips

WINE RED   PILLAR-BOX RED   SHOCKING PINK

Lips

BRICK RED   OYSTER PINK   SHOCKING PINK

Lips

BURGUNDY   CHESTNUT   COPPER

Shaping and shading

Here you can find out how to use shader, highlighter and blusher to make your face look more oval, and show off your best features.

It is best to wear shader and highlighter in the evenings. They can look too obvious during the day.

The key below shows you exactly where to put your highlighter, shader and blusher. Blend them in well, so no hard edges show.

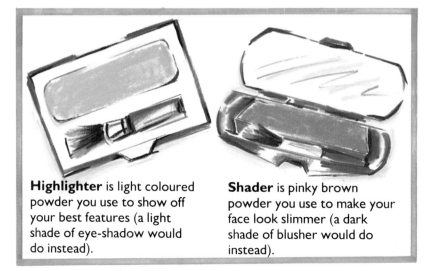

Highlighter is light coloured powder you use to show off your best features (a light shade of eye-shadow would do instead).

Shader is pinky brown powder you use to make your face look slimmer (a dark shade of blusher would do instead).

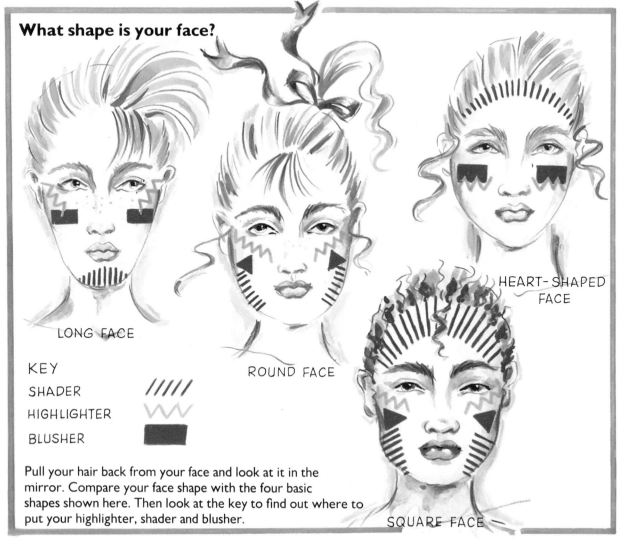

What shape is your face?

LONG FACE

ROUND FACE

HEART-SHAPED FACE

SQUARE FACE

KEY
SHADER   /////
HIGHLIGHTER   WWW
BLUSHER   ▬

Pull your hair back from your face and look at it in the mirror. Compare your face shape with the four basic shapes shown here. Then look at the key to find out where to put your highlighter, shader and blusher.

Shader

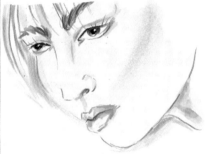

To make your cheekbones look higher, suck in your cheeks and dot shader in the hollows below them. Blend it in from your cheeks towards your hairline.

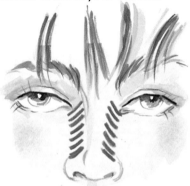

To make your nose look slimmer, dot a little shader down each side of it, or wherever your nose is uneven. Blend it in evenly with the tip of your finger.

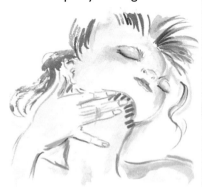

To disguise a double chin, dab a little shader just beneath your chin and blend it in well around your jawline. Make sure it does not look like a dirty tide mark.

Highlighter

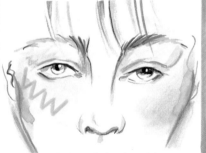

To highlight high cheekbones, dot a little highlighter just above your cheekbones and blend it in evenly, so it slants upwards towards your hairline.

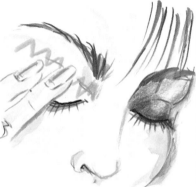

If you have attractive eyes, dab a little highlighter on to each browbone (the area just beneath your eyebrows). Blend it in so that it barely shows.

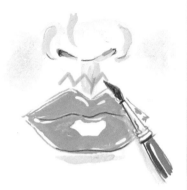

If your mouth is your best feature, use a lip brush to stroke a little highlighter into the dimple above your top lip. Blend it in evenly so it barely shows.

Blusher

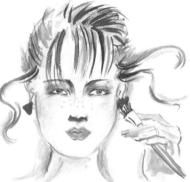

You can use blusher to give your face a better shape, as well as to give it colour. Blend it in to your highlighter and shader so that no hard lines show.

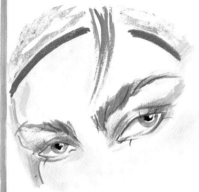

To give a hint of colour to your whole face, dot a little blusher on to each earlobe, as shown. Then blend it in well with your brush, so it barely shows.

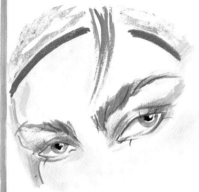

If you are looking pale, dab a little blusher around your hairline, as shown. Then blend it in thoroughly so there is just a hint of colour showing.

13

Step-by-step to a perfect make-up

Getting ready

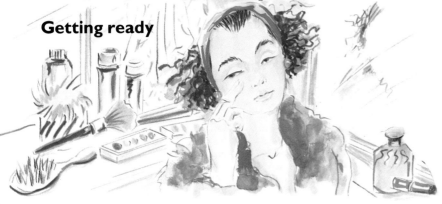

Put your make-up on in a room with a good-sized mirror and lots of light. You can find out what make-up you need on pages 8-9.

Tie your hair out of the way, or put on a headband. Wash your face and put on moisturiser. Now you are ready to begin.

Concealer

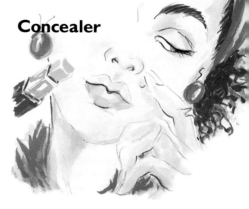

Dot a little concealer over any spots, blemishes or dark shadows and blend it in well with the tip of your finger.

Foundation

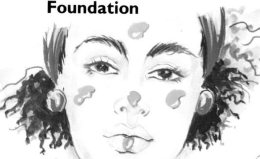

Dot a little foundation over your face. Put it over your lips too, but not your eyelids, as it will make them oily.

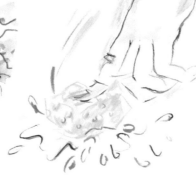

Wet your cosmetic sponge in warm water, then squeeze most of the water out and blot it on a piece of tissue.

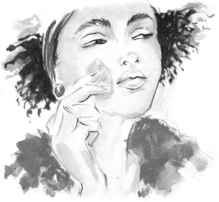

Use the sponge to spread the foundation evenly over your face. Make sure you smooth it in well under your chin.

Powder

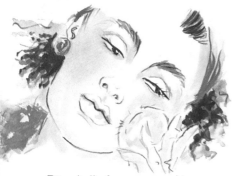

Dip a ball of cotton wool into your tub of loose powder, then pat it firmly, but gently all over your face until it is evenly covered.

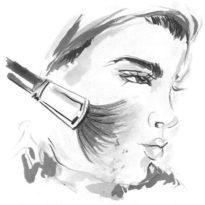

Use a large, soft powder brush to flick off the spare powder. Brush it downwards to make the tiny hairs on your face lie flat.

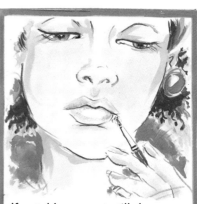

If a stubborn spot still shows through foundation and powder, dab a clean brush on your concealer and paint it out.

Blusher

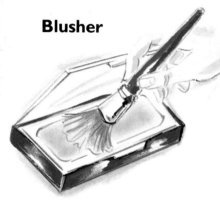

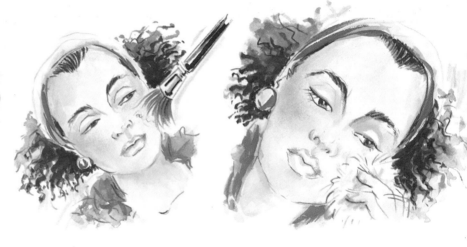

Stroke your blusher brush across your palette of powder blusher until it is lightly, but evenly, coated with powder.

Brush the blusher on to your cheekbones (this is the area just above your cheeks), and right up to your hairline.

Keep adding more until the colour is strong enough. If it starts to look too obvious, you can tone it down with powder.

Professional make-up tips

To find out what colour blusher you need, lightly pinch the skin on your cheeks. The colour which appears is the shade of blusher you need.

◆

Do not put your make-up on straight after a bath or shower as your skin is more flushed than usual. Wait until it cools down and returns to normal.

◆

You can re-cycle old lipstick ends by heating them in a bowl over a pan of boiling water. Put the mixture in a pot to go solid. Put it on with a brush.

◆

To make your eyelashes look extra thick, dust them with face powder then brush away the excess, before you put on your mascara.

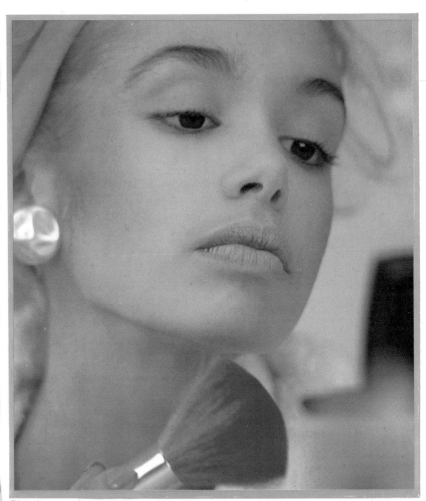

Check your finished face make-up to make sure there are no hard lines of colour anywhere.

If you can see any, blend them in with a brush. Now you are ready to make up your eyes and lips.

Eyes

Eye-shadow

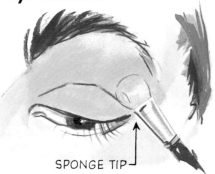

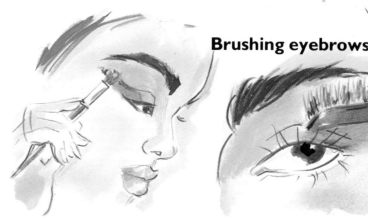

Start by stroking the lighter shade of eye-shadow over your eyelids, as shown. Blend it in with an eye-shadow brush.

Stroke the darker shade of eye-shadow on to the outer half of your eyelids, as shown. Blend in the edges with another brush.

Brushing eyebrows

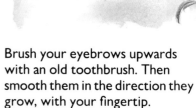

Brush your eyebrows upwards with an old toothbrush. Then smooth them in the direction they grow, with your fingertip.

Eye pencil

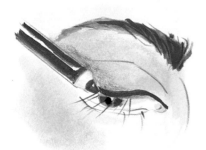

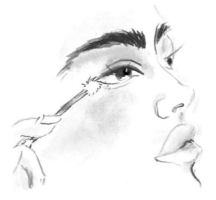

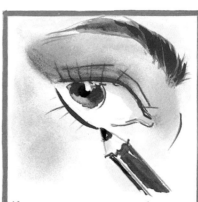

Draw a fine pencil line along your eyelids, next to your lashes, as shown. Smudge the line slightly with a damp cotton bud.

Draw another line underneath your eyes, close to your lower lashes, as shown, and smudge it gently, as before.

If you want to put pencil on the inner rim of your eye, use one which is not too sharp and draw it on carefully.

Curling eyelashes

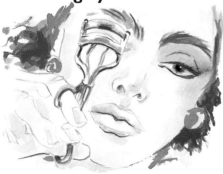

Clamp the eyelash curlers round your top lashes very carefully. Hold them shut for a minute, then open them again.

Mascara

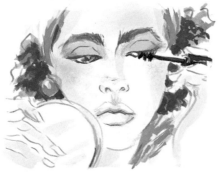

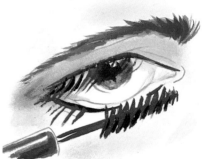

Look into a hand mirror, held at chin level. Brush mascara on to your top lashes. Let it dry, then put on a second coat.

Look straight ahead into your make-up mirror to put mascara on your bottom lashes. You only need to put on one coat.

16

Lips

Outlining your lips

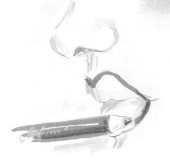

Draw an outline around the edge of your mouth with a lip pencil, resting your little finger on your chin to steady your hand.

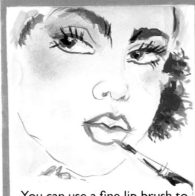

You can use a fine lip brush to outline your mouth, if you want. Dab it on your lipstick, then paint in the outline.

Putting on lipstick

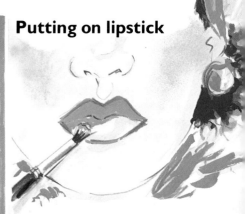

Coat your lip brush with colour from your lipstick. Carefully paint the colour on to your lips, keeping within the outline.

Blotting your lipstick

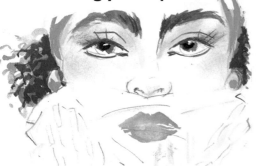

Blot your lipstick on a tissue (taking care not to smudge it). Then put on a second coat and blot your lips again.

Lip gloss

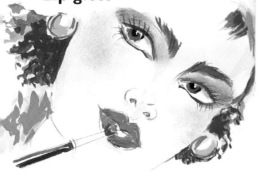

To give your lips some shine, dot lip gloss in the centre of your lips and carefully brush it outwards towards the edges.

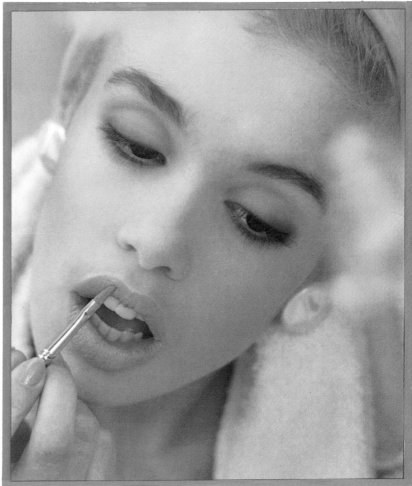

This make-up is good for evenings, when you want to make a special effort to look good.

Allow plenty of time to do it. You can see how to do a quick, simple make-up over the page.

The natural look

All you need for a simple, natural looking make-up are the things shown here.

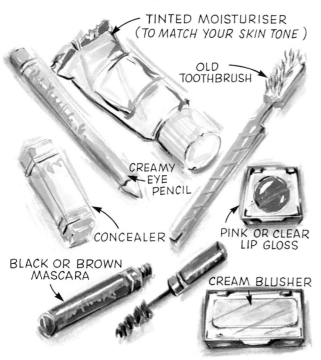

TINTED MOISTURISER
(TO MATCH YOUR SKIN TONE)

OLD TOOTHBRUSH

CREAMY EYE PENCIL

CONCEALER

PINK OR CLEAR LIP GLOSS

BLACK OR BROWN MASCARA

CREAM BLUSHER

1 Concealer and tinted moisturiser

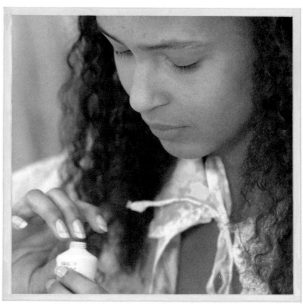

Tie your hair back. Wash your face and pat it dry. Cover any blemishes with concealer (see page 14). Dot moisturiser on with your finger and smooth it in.

2 Blusher

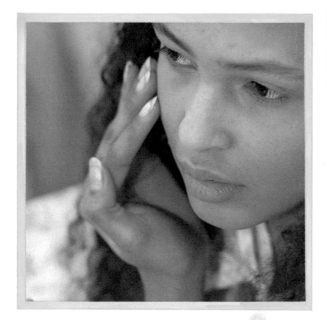

Use your fingertips to dot blusher on to your cheeks, then carefully smooth the blusher outwards and upwards towards your hairline.

3 Eye pencil

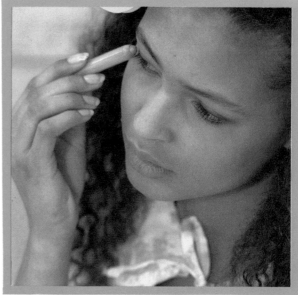

Carefully draw a pencil line across your eyelid, next to your eyelashes. Then smooth the colour over your eyelid, using a damp cotton bud, or your fingertip.

4   Mascara

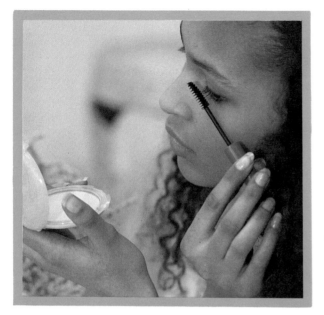

Brush mascara on to your upper lashes, as on page 16, let it dry and then apply a second coat. Brush one coat of mascara on to your lower lashes.

5   Brushing your eyebrows

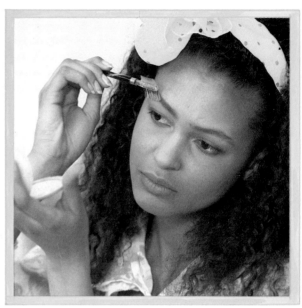

Use an old toothbrush to brush your eyebrows upwards. Then wet your finger and smooth it over each eyebrow in the direction it grows.

6   Lip gloss

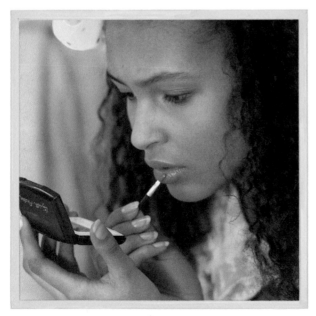

Using a lip brush, paint lip gloss carefully on to your lips. Do not brush it right to the edge of your mouth, as it can 'run' and look rather messy.

7   The finished look

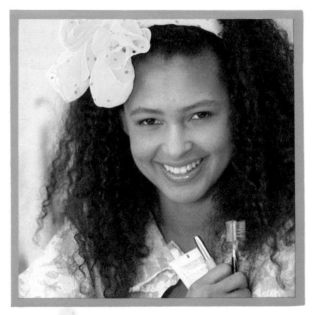

This is what the finished make-up should look like. With a bit of practise, you will be able to do it in a matter of minutes.

Top-to-toe beauty routine

If you are planning a special night out and want to look and feel your best, give yourself an all-over beauty treatment, following this step-by-step plan.

Set aside a few hours (you will need at least two) so that you can relax and really enjoy yourself. If you are going out with a friend, you could ask her over so you can have fun getting ready together.

Having a bath

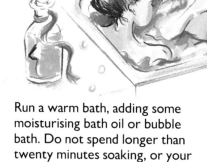

Run a warm bath, adding some moisturising bath oil or bubble bath. Do not spend longer than twenty minutes soaking, or your skin will start to wrinkle.

While you are in the bath, take a handful of coarse sea salt and rub it over your bottom and thighs to stimulate your circulation and make you tingle.

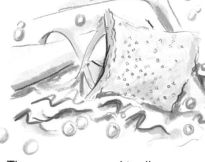

Then massage your skin all over with a textured bath mitt. Its rough surface will rub off any dead skin and leave your body feeling soft and smooth.

Get out of the bath and pat yourself dry with a soft towel. Dust some talc over your feet and under your arms (use deodorant under your arms, if you prefer).

Massage a moisturising body lotion all your body (if your skin is dry, use body oil). Pay special attention to dry skin on your heels and elbows.

Conditioning your hair

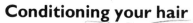
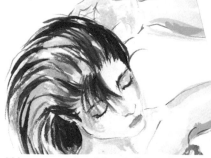

Warm two mugfuls of olive oil or almond oil in a saucepan (do not let it get too hot, or it will scald you). Massage it into your hair until it is all absorbed.

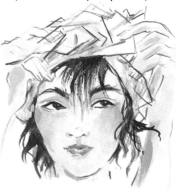

Wrap a piece of clingfilm around your hair, overlapping it at the front. Scrunch it up to seal the ends together. Make sure you do not drip oil on your clothes.

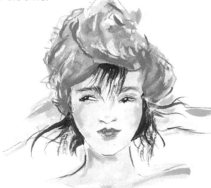

Then wrap a warm towel round your head in a turban. Leave it on for thirty minutes. You can see how to wash out the oil on the next page.

Putting on a face mask

While your hair conditioner is working, put on a face mask (see below for recipes). You can find out how to do this on page 7.

You can put thin slices of cucumber or potato on your eyes if you like. This soothes them.

Put on some soothing music, lie back and relax for ten minutes. Then rinse off the face mask with warm water and pat your face dry with a soft towel.

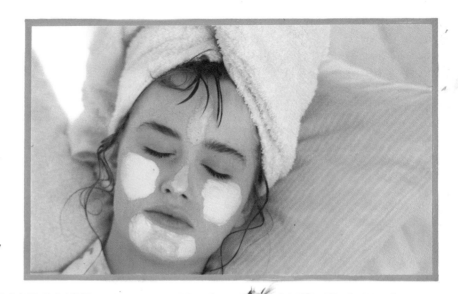

Home-made face masks

For dry skin: mix together a tablespoon of plain yogurt, a teaspoon of runny honey and a mashed, ripe avocado. Spread the mixture on your face and leave it on for ten to fifteen minutes.

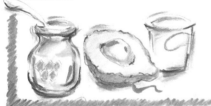

For oily skin: mix together a tablespoon of plain yogurt, a teaspoon of honey, a teaspoon of oatmeal and a mashed peach. Spread it on your face and leave for ten minutes.

For normal skin: crush a few thick slices of cucumber to a pulp and mix them with a teaspoon of plain yogurt and a few drops of rose water. Spread the mixture on your face and leave it on for fifteen minutes.

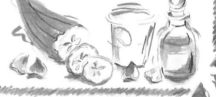

Removing unwanted hair

Everyone has hair on their legs, but there is no need to remove it unless you really want to.

Depilatory cream is the gentlest and easiest method of removing hair. It is safer than shaving and less painful than waxing your legs.

If you decide to remove the hair on your legs, it is best to remove it regularly. The hairs that grow back look thicker, because they are short and stubbly.

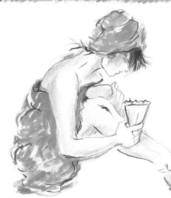

Read the instructions on the packet before you start. Squeeze some cream into the palm of your hand, then spread it thickly over your legs with your fingers.

Leave it on for as long as the packet tells you to. Then wipe it off gently with a wet cloth. Rinse your legs and then pat them dry with a towel.

Washing your hair

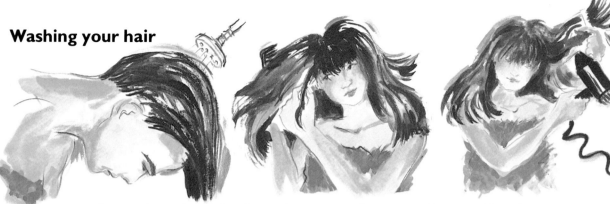

When your conditioning hair oil has been on for half an hour, wash it off. Shampoo your hair twice and rinse it thoroughly to remove every trace of the oil.

Comb your hair very gently to remove any tangles. Start at the ends of your hair and work back towards your head. Do not tug the comb through clumps of your hair.

If you are blow drying your hair, do it in sections. Hold the hair dryer at least ten cm from your hair and keep it moving, as you dry, to avoid damaging your hair.

Styling your hair

You can buy soft, fabric hair curlers like the ones in the photograph which will curl your hair without damaging it. You can make corkscrew curls or soft waves.

Put them in your hair and leave them for 45 minutes. Meanwhile you can give yourself a manicure and pedicure (see below and opposite).

When you take the curlers out, gently brush your hair, or just run your fingers through it, to separate the curls.

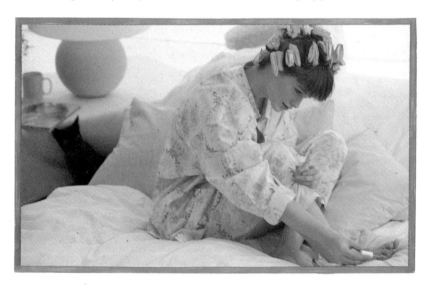

Your hands

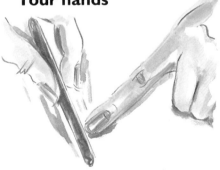
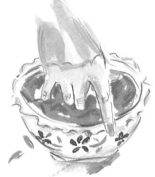
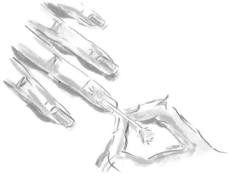

Treat your hands to a manicure before you go out. First, file your nails with an emery board. It is best to file from the edges to the centre of your nails.

Then soak your fingertips in warm, soapy water for a few minutes. If your nails are dirty, scrub them with a nailbrush. Dry your hands. Then rub on some hand cream.

Rub some cuticle cream into the hard pads of skin at the base of your nails to soften them. Then gently push back the cuticle with a cotton bud.

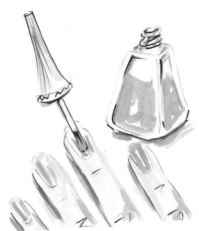

Carefully paint on a thin coat of nail varnish. There are some ideas for party nails on page 25. When the varnish is dry, carefully put on another coat.

Your feet

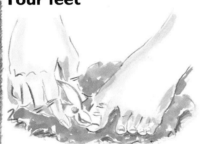

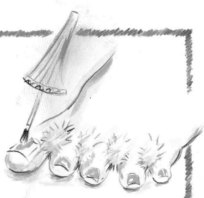

Now you can give yourself a pedicure. Trim your toenails straight across with nail clippers. Then file them from the edges inwards.

Soften your cuticles with cream and push them back. Then separate your toes with cotton wool* and put on two coats of varnish.

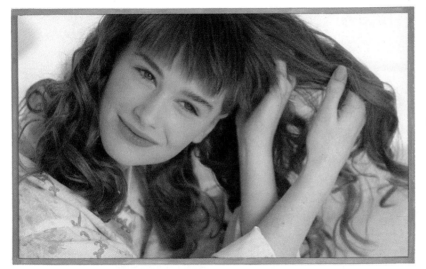

Plucking your eyebrows

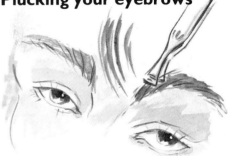

Before you put your make-up on, tidy your eyebrows by plucking any straggly hairs that grow beneath them. Pluck them in the direction they grow.

Make-up

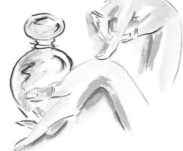

Now you can put on your make-up. First, tie your hair back and put some moisturiser on your face. Then, turn to pages 24 to 31 for some ideas on party make-up.

Scent

If you wear scent, such as toilet water or perfume, dab a little on your pulse points (behind your ears and knees and on the inside of your wrists and elbows).

Ready to go

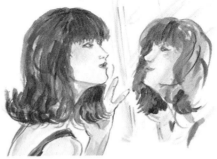

Now you can get dressed. Make sure you don't spoil your hair or smudge your make-up. Check your appearance in a full length mirror before you go out.

* You can buy foam toe pads from the chemists, which do the same thing.

23

Party make-up

Party make-up can be anything from bold eyeshadow and bright lipstick, to false eyelashes, sequins and turquoise mascara. Here are some things to collect.

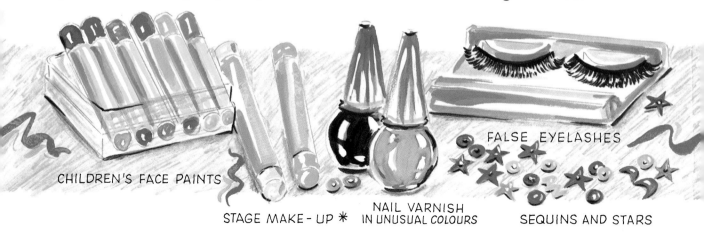

CHILDREN'S FACE PAINTS

STAGE MAKE-UP *

NAIL VARNISH IN UNUSUAL COLOURS

FALSE EYELASHES

SEQUINS AND STARS

Eye-shadows

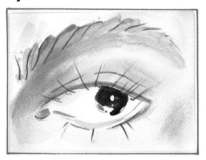

You can buy little pots of loose, sparkly powder eye-shadow in lots of colours. To stop it from spilling on to your cheeks, put it on with a damp brush.

Mascara

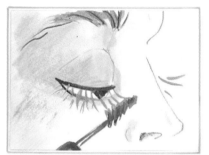

You can buy mascara in lots of bright colours, such as violet and green. If you want a hint of colour, brush it on to the tips of your lashes only.

Eyebrows

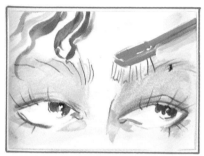

You can colour your eyebrows to match your mascara. Dab a little mascara on your eyebrow brush. Blot the brush on a tissue, then brush your eyebrows with it.

False eye-lashes

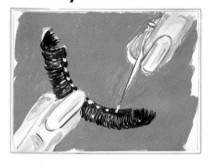

Put these on before your eye-shadow. Apply a coat of mascara, then dot eyelash glue along the lash band with a pin. Make sure you glue each end.

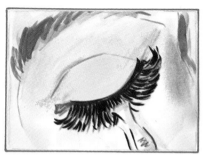

Let the glue dry for a second. Then pick up the lashes with a pair of tweezers and position them on your closed eyelid, on top of your real lashes.

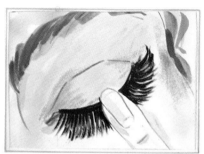

Gently press the lash band down on to your eyelid with your finger. Wait for the glue to dry, then brush the eyelashes upwards with an old toothbrush.

* If you have difficulty finding stage make-up, you can write to Charles Fox Ltd, theatre make-up suppliers, 22 Tavistock St, London WC2.

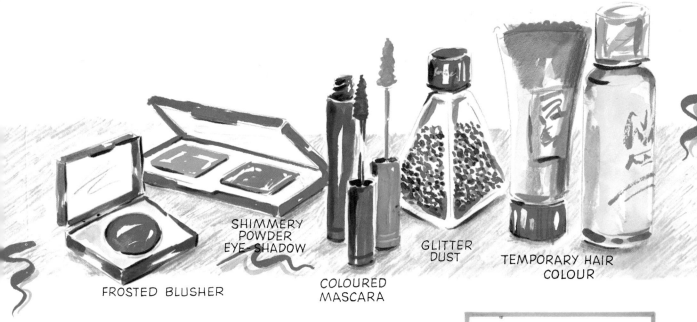

SHIMMERY POWDER EYE-SHADOW

FROSTED BLUSHER

COLOURED MASCARA

GLITTER DUST

TEMPORARY HAIR COLOUR

Designer finger nails

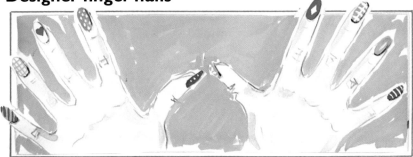

Manicure your nails as on page 22. Then put on nail varnish. You can buy it in lots of bright colours. Use two or more colours to paint on spots, stripes, checks or any design you like. If you are using more than one colour, make sure each coat is thoroughly dry before you apply the next, or your nail varnish will smudge.

Glitter dust and sequins

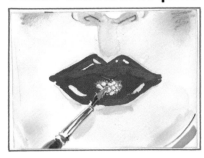

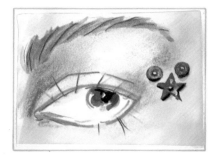

You can make shimmery lip gloss by mixing some glitter dust with your ordinary lip gloss in the palm of your hand. Then brush it on your lips, in the usual way.

Add shine to your make-up by glueing sequins on your face with eyelash glue. Put them at the outer corners of your eyes, or glue one on as a beauty spot.

Colouring your hair

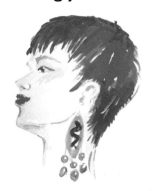

You can change your hair colour for the evening, using a wash in/wash out hair colour mousse or shampoo, in an unusual colour.

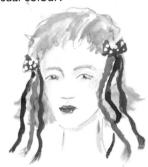

Another way of adding flashes of colour to your hair, is to attach thin swatches of false hair to your own, using slides or ribbons.

Polka dot make-up

This party make-up combines the sophistication of black and white with the fun of polka dots for a stunning effect.

You will need

light beige foundation
translucent powder
white and dark grey powder eye-
  shadows
black eye pencil
black mascara
pale pink or white lipstick
matching lip pencil

Foundation

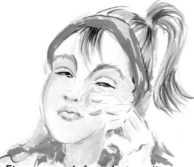

First, smooth foundation all over your face and neck, using a cosmetic sponge. You can check the techniques for applying this make-up, on pages 14-17.

Powder

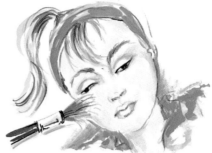

Then powder your face quite thickly using a cotton wool ball, or a powder puff and gently flick off any spare powder with your powder brush.

Eye-shadow

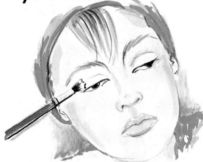

Brush a thick layer of white eye-shadow over the whole of your eyelid, as shown. You may need two coats to get the heavy, matt effect shown here.

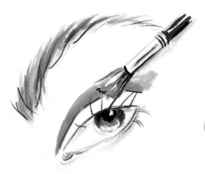

Then brush dark grey eye-shadow along the line of your eye socket as shown, broadening the line towards the outer corner of your eye. Blend it in with a brush.

Eye pencil

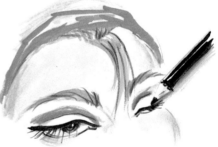

Carefully draw a fine black pencil line along your eyelid, close to your upper eyelashes. Then smudge it slightly with a damp cotton bud, or your finger.

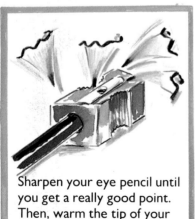

Sharpen your eye pencil until you get a really good point. Then, warm the tip of your pencil in the palm of your hand, so it goes on thickly.

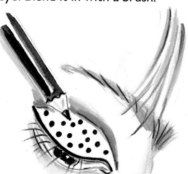

Draw pencil dots on your eyelids, as shown. Press firmly but gently with the tip of the pencil, turning it slightly at the same time, so the dots show up well.

Mascara

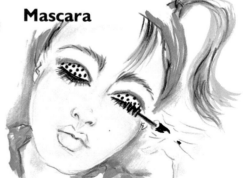

Curl your eyelashes with eyelash curlers, then brush mascara on to your upper lashes. Let it dry, then put on a second coat. Put one coat on your lower lashes.

Brushing eyebrows

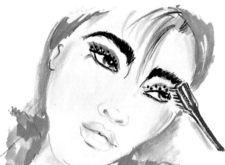

Brush your eyebrows with your eyebrow brush. Then dip the tip of your finger in a little Vaseline and smooth it over your eyebrows to make them shine.

Lipstick

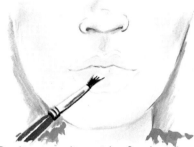

Outline your lips with a fine brush, or a lip pencil which matches your lipstick. Then put on your lipstick. Blot it on a tissue, apply another coat and blot again.

Too pale?

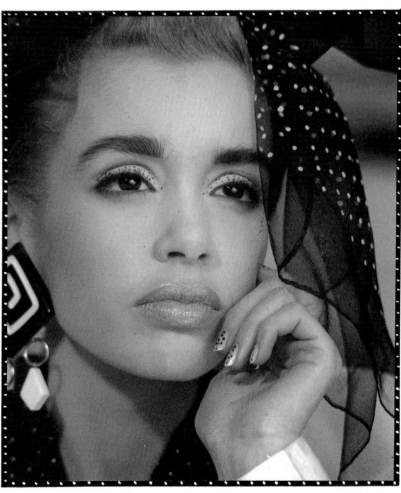

If you think your finished make-up looks too pale, brush on a little pink blusher. Make sure you blend it in well.

Hair

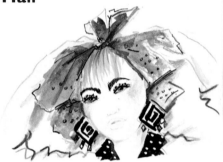

If you have short hair, smooth it back with hair gel. If your hair is long, tie it back, then tie a scarf round your head in a big, floppy bow, as shown.

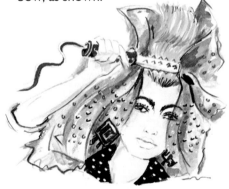

If you have a fringe, put setting lotion on it, then use curling tongs to make it wavy. Comb it upwards and spray hair spray on it to make it stand up.

Wear black and white clothes with this look, for maximum effect.

There is another, quite different party make-up on the next page.

Razzle dazzle make-up

You are sure to be noticed in this colourful party make-up. You can use different colours from the ones shown here if you like.

You will need

foundation
translucent powder
golden peach blusher
orange, sea green and smoky
  grey eye-shadows
black and emerald green mascara
orange lipstick
matching lip pencil and lip brush
gold lip gloss

Foundation

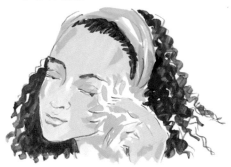

First, smooth foundation all over your face and neck, using a cosmetic sponge. You can check the techniques for putting on make-up on pages 14-17.

Powder

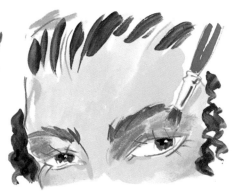

Then powder your face lightly all over, using a cotton wool ball or a powder puff. Gently flick off any loose powder with your powder brush.

Blusher

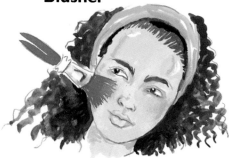

Brush blusher on to your cheeks, as shown. You can put on a little more in the evening than you would during the day, but make sure you blend it in well.

Eye-shadow

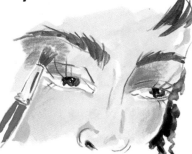

Brush orange eye-shadow on to the inner half of one eyelid and the outer half of the other eyelid. You can put on quite a lot, as long as you blend it in well.

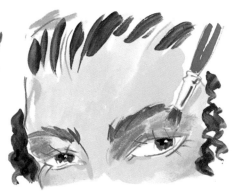

Brush green eye-shadow on to the other half of each eyelid and blend it in well where it meets the orange eyeshadow, so that the two colours merge.

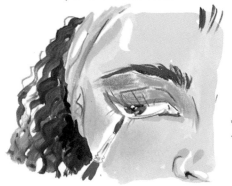

Dampen a fine tipped brush and use it to stroke grey eye-shadow in a fine line along your upper lash line and at the outer corners of the lower lashes.

Mascara

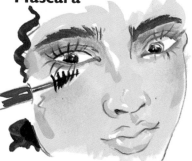

Brush black mascara on to your upper and lower eye lashes (you can see how on page 16). When it is dry, brush a second coat on your upper lashes.

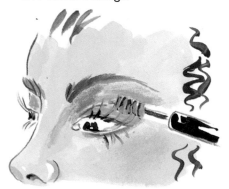

Brush emerald green mascara carefully on to the tips of your eyelashes. If you want a stronger shade of green, wait for it to dry, then put on a second coat.

Brushing eyebrows

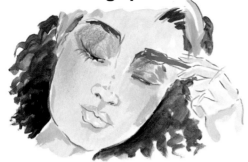

Brush your eyebrows upwards (you can put a little brown eye-shadow on the brush if you want to darken them). Then smooth them with your finger.

Lipstick

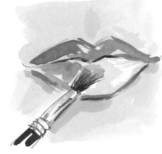

Outline your lips with your orange lip pencil (or a lip brush coated with lipstick). Fill in the colour with your orange lipstick and a lip brush keeping within the outline.

Lip gloss

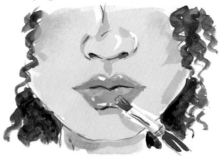

Brush a little gold lip gloss on to the middle of your lower lip to make your lips look fuller. You could use non-toxic gold eye-shadow instead.

Hair

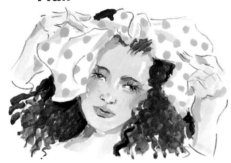

If you have long hair which is not naturally curly, curl it as on page 22. Then tie a brightly coloured scarf round your head in a big, floppy bow.

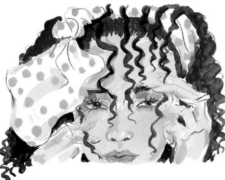

If you have a fringe, pull a few wispy strands of it down in front of your eyes and then gently finger a little hair gel through it to separate the curls.

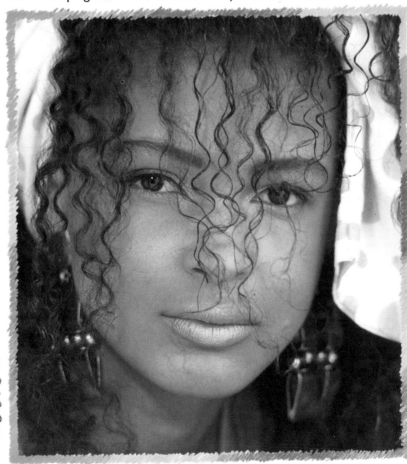

You can match your eyeshadow colours with the clothes you are going to wear.

Try unusual colour combinations, such as orange and pink, or yellow and blue.

Four nostalgic looks

Here you can find out how to create some distinctive make-up looks from the twenties, forties, fifties and sixties.

You can dress the part, too, whether it's for a special party with a nostalgic theme, or just for fun.

The 1920s

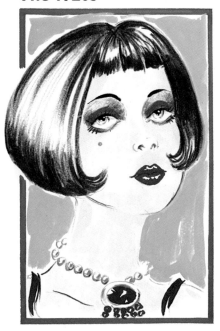

In the 1920s girls wore bold eye make-up, bright lipstick and sometimes a false beauty spot. They often had their hair bobbed.

You will need: pale foundation, translucent powder, dark eye-shadow, black mascara, dark eyebrow pencil, glossy pink or red lipstick and a matching lip pencil or lip brush.

Face: put on your foundation and powder.

Eyes: brush eye-shadow over your eyelids and browbones. Smudge a little under your lower lashes. Then put on lots of mascara. Pencil in narrow, arched eyebrows.

Lips: were painted in a very distinctive shape in the twenties. Outline them with lip pencil to emphasize your 'Cupid's Bow' (the dimple in your top lip). Then put on your lipstick, being careful to keep within the outline.

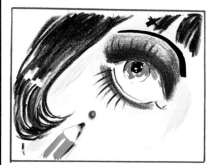

Finally, paint or stick on a false beauty spot, as shown.

The 1940s

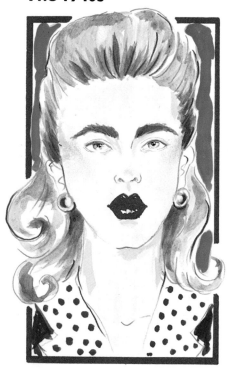

Make-up was bold and glamorous in the 1940s. Girls painted on dark eyebrows and bright red lips. They often wore their hair elegantly rolled at the front, and left the back loose round their shoulders.

You will need: pale foundation, translucent powder, dark blusher (in brown or plum), grey or brown eye pencil, eyebrow pencil, glossy red lipstick and matching lip pencil, or a lip brush.

Face: put on your foundation and powder. Brush blusher high on your cheekbones.

Eyes: brush eye-shadow on your eyelids, close to your eyelashes. Put mascara on your top lashes only. Thicken and darken your eyebrows with eyebrow pencil.

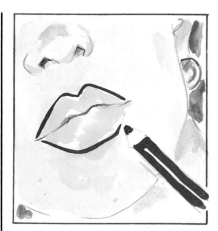

Lips: outline them carefully with your lip pencil, squaring off the bottom lip slightly, as shown. Then paint them with two or three coats of lipstick, keeping within the outline. Blot your lips between each coat, so your lipstick will stay on longer.

The 1950s

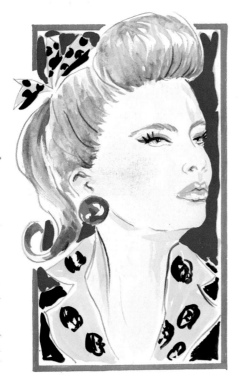

Fifties make-up concentrated on the eyes. Black eyeliner swept up at the corners gave eyes a cat-like look. Girls wore their hair in high pony tails, with the front rolled, or worn in a short, neat fringe.

You will need: light beige foundation, slightly lighter powder, pink blusher, light blue or yellow eye-shadow, liquid eyeliner, a few false eyelashes, eyelash glue, mascara, pink lip pencil and pale pink pearly lipstick.

Face: put on your foundation, powder and blusher.

Eyes: brush eye-shadow on to your eyelids. Carefully paint a narrow line of liquid eyeliner close to your top eyelashes, winging it upwards slightly at the outer corners of your eyes.

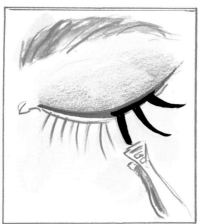

Cut small sections off complete false eyelashes and stick them at the outer corners of your eyes with eyelash glue, as shown. Brush two coats of mascara on to your upper lashes only.

Lips: outline them with lip pencil and fill in with lipstick.

The 1960s

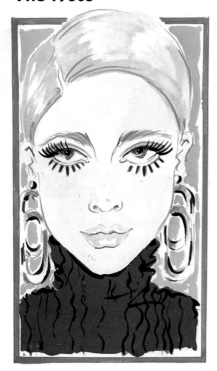

Girls in the 1960s wore a lot of dark eye make-up. Faces and lips were as pale as possible. Girls wore their hair in short, boyish haircuts, or backcombed into a glamorous 'bouffant' style.

You will need: pale foundation and powder, pale matt eye-shadow (pink or white), grey eye pencil, black liquid eyeliner, false eyelashes, eyelash glue, black eye pencil, black mascara, pale matt lipstick.

Face: put on your foundation and powder.

Eyes: brush on your eye-shadow. Draw a thickish line of grey eye pencil along the rim of your socket and smudge it slightly. Then, paint a line of liquid eyeliner along your top eyelashes.

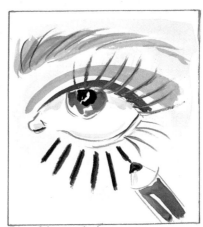

Glue false eyelashes on to your upper eyelids (see page 24 for the method). Then draw in false eyelashes underneath your eyes with black eye pencil. Put on several coats of mascara.

Lips: cover them with foundation, then put on your lipstick.

31

Index

Acknowledgements

photographer **Simon Bottomley**
session co-ordinator **Saskia Sarginson**
stylist **Sara Sarre**
make-up and hair **Louise Constad**
hair, pages 18-19, 15, 17, 27 **Tony Collins** for Joshua Galvin
models **Mickey** at Synchro, **Akure** at Look, **Emma Campbell** and **Louise Kelly** at Select

The following companies kindly contributed clothes and accessories for the photographs:

Liberty, Goldie, Fenwicks, Corocraft, Katharine Glazier and Extras (both at Hyper, Hyper), Alexis Lahellec, Oui, Hyper Hyper, Molton Brown.
All room sets from Habitat

With thanks to:
Rosemary Ross and pupils of St Paul's Girls School, Brook Green, London W6.

Sandra Nikpour and pupils of Highbury Hill High School, Highbury Hill, London N5.

The following organizations kindly gave permission to reproduce the photographs on these pages:

page 10 left, Elle/Transworld
page 10 right and centre, and page 11 right, Jacinte/Transworld
page 11 left, Fashion Fair
page 11 centre, Seventeen at Boots

First published in 1986 by Usborne Publishing Ltd, 20 Garrick Street, London WC2E 9BJ, England.
Copyright © 1986 Usborne Publishing Ltd.

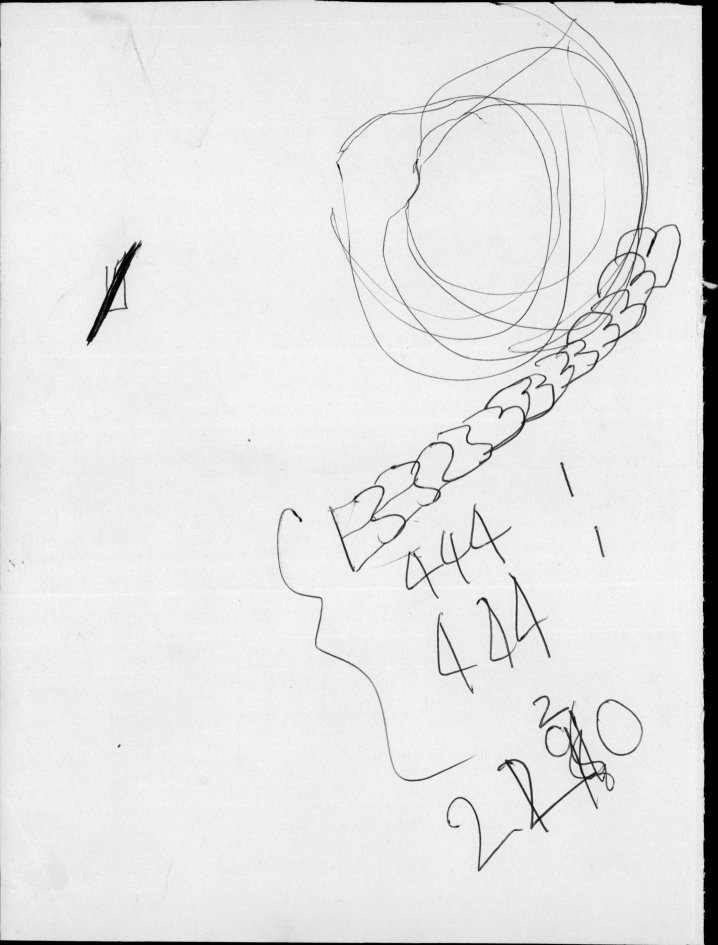